Mealtime Mindset

How Changing Your Mindset Changes Mealtimes

by
Christine Miroddi Yoder

Founder of Foodology Feeding · Creator of the Mealtime Mindset™ Framework

SECOND EDITION
Completely revised and expanded.

For Luke and Ava.

Contents

Before We Begin

Over the years, my understanding of pediatric feeding has continued to evolve. Today I teach what I call The Four Pillars of Feeding:

- Gut Health
- Sensory Processing (including nervous system regulation)
- Oral Motor Skills
- Mindset

Together, these four pillars provide a framework for understanding why children struggle with eating and how to help them make lasting progress.

This book focuses on one pillar: Mindset.

Why?

Because regardless of whether your child's feeding challenges stem from gut health, sensory processing, oral motor skills, or a combination of all three, the emotional environment surrounding food matters. Every child benefits from mealtimes built on trust, safety, consistency, and connection.

Think of this book as your guide to strengthening the Mindset Pillar. Once you've built this foundation, you'll be better prepared to understand and support the other pillars of feeding as well.

Introduction

If you're holding this book, chances are mealtimes have become stressful. Maybe you've made separate meals, negotiated one more bite, worried your child isn't eating enough, or ended dinner feeling defeated. If that's you, I want you to know something before we begin:

There is hope—and there is a path forward.

More importantly, there is a reason your family ended up here.

And it's probably not because you're doing anything wrong. Most parents aren't failing. They've been given a puzzle to solve with missing pieces and no picture on the box. At least that's how I felt when I started putting these pieces together!

I'm Christine Miroddi Yoder, pediatric feeding specialist, founder of Foodology Feeding, and creator of the Mealtime Mindset™ framework. For years I've helped families whose children eat only a handful of foods, gag at the table, melt down during meals, or seem terrified of trying something new. I've also lived this journey as a parent.

Before we dive in, I have one request.

Your Free Companion Workbook

I've created a free companion workbook to help you as you go through this book.

Throughout these pages, I'll ask you to reflect, write, and apply what you're learning. The workbook gives you space to turn these ideas into action so you can create real change in your home.

Scan the code below to download your free copy of The Mealtime Mindset Companion Workbook:

Scan to download

Don't skip this step. The more you engage with the exercises, the more you'll get from this book.

*A confident eater isn't built
one bite at a time.*

*They're built one positive
mealtime at a time.*

PART I

Change Your Perspective

Before we can change what happens at the table, we have to change the way we see it.

CHAPTER ONE

It Doesn't Start With Food

If you had met me early in my career, you probably would have thought I was a good feeding therapist.

I followed the training I had been given. I measured success by compliance. How many bites did the child take? Did they move from looking at the food to touching it? From touching it to licking it? Did they complete the task I asked them to do?

Those were the goals.

Parents often waited outside the therapy room while I worked one-on-one with their child. We celebrated measurable progress, and many children did improve. At the time, I genuinely believed I was helping.

Looking back, I realize something was missing.

The children were learning how to comply.

They weren't necessarily learning how to enjoy food.

They weren't building positive memories around the dinner table.

Food wasn't becoming something they looked forward to—it was becoming another task to complete.

I didn't know there was another way because I had never been taught another way.

Then my thinking began to change.

As I continued my education, I was introduced to approaches that asked different questions. Instead of focusing only on what a child did with food, they challenged me to think about how a child felt about food. Around that same time, life gave me an even greater teacher than any course ever could—I became a mother.

When my own son struggled with feeding, everything became personal.

Suddenly, I wasn't just looking at data sheets and therapy goals. I was sitting at my own dinner table wondering if my child would eat. I experienced the worry, the frustration, the second-guessing, and the deep desire every parent has to simply enjoy a meal with their family.

That's when my biggest realization happened.

I had spent years measuring bites.

But bites weren't the goal.

The real goal was helping children feel safe enough, confident enough, and curious enough to enjoy food—not just during therapy, but for the rest of their lives.

That realization changed everything.

From that day forward, I couldn't look at feeding therapy the same way.

I stopped celebrating compliance.

I started celebrating curiosity.

I stopped asking, "How many bites?"

I started asking, "How did that child feel at the table today?"

Every therapy goal began to change.

It changed the way I practiced. It changed the way I coached parents. It changed the goals I wrote, the words I used, and the way I measured success.

But perhaps most importantly, it changed where I started.

Like many parents, I used to think feeding therapy started with food.

It doesn't start with food.

Over the years, working with hundreds of families, continuing my education, challenging my own assumptions, and doing my own inner work, I began to notice patterns. The families who made the greatest progress didn't necessarily have the easiest children. They had the strongest foundation.

Before we worried about trying another food, we worked on our Mealtime Mindset.

Before we asked a child to taste broccoli, we established clear boundaries and Mealtime Agreements.

Before we expected progress, we created safety, trust, and consistency.

I watched families come to us after unsuccessful hospital programs, feeding therapy, well-meaning advice from friends and relatives, and years of trial and error. Nearly all of them had one thing in common.

It's kind of like if you were to hire a contractor to build the second floor of your house before pouring the foundation. They were trying to build the second story of a house that didn't yet have a foundation. Yet that's what many feeding approaches unintentionally ask families to do. They start with the food before they've built the foundation that allows change to last.

Every new strategy eventually came crashing down—not because the family wasn't trying hard enough, but because they had skipped the first and most important step.

So I began organizing everything I had learned into a framework.

Not just from one course.

Not just from one mentor.

But from years of clinical experience, continuing education, raising my own family, learning from the families I served, and continually refining my own thinking.

Over time, those lessons became a repeatable framework that I now teach every family before we ever focus on expanding foods.

I call it Mealtime Mindset.

The ideas you're about to learn aren't random tips or isolated strategies. They are the foundation I now build with every family before we ever focus on expanding foods. This is the exact framework we teach and coach and hold our parents' hands through in our signature program Unlocking Mealtimes.

Because once the foundation is strong, everything else becomes easier to build.

And like any good framework, it continues to evolve. As I continue learning, researching, and serving families, I expect my understanding to grow. But one thing has remained constant:

Children learn best when they feel safe.

Families make the greatest progress when everyone is working from the same foundation.

That's the foundation I'm honored to share with you in this book.

My Promise to You

I can't promise your child will love broccoli next week.

I can't promise dinner will magically become peaceful overnight.

But I can promise this:

If you build the right foundation first, you'll stop feeling like you're fighting food every single day.

That's why I wrote this book.

I'm going to do my best to give you the clearest and most compelling arguments to shift your mindset around food and meals. First, I will ask you to make four commitments so you get the best results.

The Four Commitments

COMMITMENT 1

I will trade pressure for progress.

If you remember only one thing from this book, let it be this: pressure may get a bite today, but it often steals progress tomorrow. From this point forward, we're measuring success differently. We're looking for curiosity, comfort, confidence, and connection—not just bites.

COMMITMENT 2

I will be consistent.

Consistency doesn't mean being perfect. It means showing up again tomorrow. It means using the same language, the same expectations, and the same approach across caregivers whenever possible. Children learn through repetition, and lasting progress comes from hundreds of small moments—not one perfect meal.

I will trust the process.

There isn't a magical strategy hidden in Chapter 9 that suddenly changes everything overnight. Real progress happens through hundreds of small, positive experiences with food.

I will become a student of my child.

From this point forward, I'd like you to become a student of your child. Instead of asking, "Why won't they just eat?" begin asking different questions:

> *What is my child trying to communicate?*
>
> *What feels unsafe about this food?*
>
> *What skill might they be missing?*
>
> *What belief have they developed around eating?*

The quality of the questions you ask determines the quality of the answers you find. Curious parents become great problem solvers—and great problem solvers help children make lasting progress.

Knowledge Isn't Enough—Action Is

These commitments alone aren't enough. You can think about it and talk about what to do all day long, but if you don't apply the strategies in this book, no amount of knowledge you have will produce the changes you're looking for!

As you read a book, you take in a lot of information, and if you're dedicated to finding the answers and seeing progress, you will implement what you learn and see amazing changes. But what I often see is people start off very motivated, and then life gets in the way, and then they forget to implement—or they had a rough day of their child whining and throwing a tantrum about food, so you put it off, and sometimes people just give up altogether. It's easy to chase the next gadget, supplement, social media tip, or miracle program promising to fix picky eating overnight. Don't go down that path! Follow the plan and the strategies outlined in this book. If you follow the strategies, if you implement them and really make an effort to change your mindset and your child's mindset, you will see improvement week by week. It really needs to be consistent though!

Many of you will be learning these principles for the very first time; for others, there will be ideas you have heard before or read about or watched a video on. It may be presented here with a new slant, or I may help you reach a new level of understanding.

Throughout the pages of this book, you will learn to master the fundamentals, and if you apply them, over and over, you will see your child achieve success with food. You will find both practical steps and principles of mindset that will improve mealtimes for you and your child—and that will stay with you both for a lifetime.

So, if you are serious about your child's eating, you need to take mealtime seriously! You can't just desire for it to happen without putting in the action steps. You can see success, but you have to make it a priority. If you think about and focus on sports and work, that is what will take priority and that is what you will see progress with. If the focus of your mind is on food and mealtimes, that is where you will see success happen. But you really can't always have both.

For example, I had a client who wanted so badly for their child to read. We made an appointment and I went to their house after school, and she said, "Oh sorry, we have to leave to go to tennis—we can only do a half hour." I asked her to take him to the local library and spend 30 minutes in the children's section having him look at books, and to take home ANY book that looked remotely interesting to him. She never went all summer. Reading success was what she desired, but it wasn't where her mind was, and it wasn't her priority. She told me that through her actions—or really, her lack of action! We all make time for what we truly believe matters. If feeding is important to you, it deserves more than good intentions—it deserves consistent action.

I will give you the tools, but if you are not consistent and don't use them, the outcome won't change.

On the flip side, when you do put in the time, the results are incredible! One of my favorite feeding clients was so dedicated! She didn't miss a session and implemented everything I asked. She even did the Safe and Sound Protocol and went to the recommended specialists I thought would be beneficial. I asked her to try cooking the same meal we made during the week (eggs and guacamole), and then to build and use one of those foods in another meal during the week. Well, she texted me not three days later telling me he ate guacamole and chips that day! Success! Over the course of about a year, he learned to drink from an open cup, drink from a straw, do a proper rotary chew, and added about 35 new foods to his repertoire. Those are the shifts I am talking about. It was her dedication to his success and the action steps she took to move him forward that allowed him to be so successful. She trusted the process. She followed through with every recommendation, practiced consistently at home, and kept showing up.

That is the progress I want for you too!

> ## Key Takeaways
>
> - Positive mealtime experiences are the foundation for lasting feeding success.
>
> - Progress begins with mindset—not with another bite.
>
> - Pressure may get a bite today, but it often steals progress tomorrow.
>
> - A strong foundation of trust, consistency, and clear mealtime agreements makes every other feeding strategy more effective.

*A confident eater isn't built
one bite at a time.*

*They're built one positive
mealtime at a time.*

. . .

CHAPTER TWO

When Food Stops Feeling Safe

"Ew."

"Yuck."

"No!"

"I don't like it."

"That's Mommy's food."

"Gross!"

If you're reading this book, you've probably heard at least one of those phrases. Maybe you've heard all of them.

But I want you to pause for a moment and think back.

Was your child always this way?

Can you remember a time when they happily explored new foods? Maybe they reached for whatever was on your plate. Maybe they smiled while trying something new. Or perhaps feeding has been challenging from the very beginning.

Whatever your story looks like, I want you to know something.

Your child didn't wake up one morning and decide to become "picky."

Children don't refuse food because they're trying to make our lives difficult.

They're communicating.

The challenge is that most of the time, they don't yet have the words to tell us what they're trying to say.

As parents, we naturally see the behavior.

They push the plate away.

Turn their head.

Throw the food.

Cry.

Clamp their mouth shut.

We see the behavior...

...but we don't always see what created it.

One of the biggest mindset shifts you'll make throughout this book is learning to ask a different question.

Instead of asking:

"Why won't my child eat?"

begin asking:

"What is my child trying to communicate?"

That one question changes everything.

Food Is Never Just Food

Food is emotional.

Long before I became a feeding specialist, food was tied to memories, traditions, celebrations, comfort, and family.

I'd imagine that's true for you too.

Think back to one of your earliest positive food memories.

Was it baking cookies with your grandmother?

A favorite birthday cake?

Ice cream after little league?

Sunday dinner with your family?

Write it down.

Food:

Feeling:

Now think about a food memory that wasn't so positive.

Maybe you became sick after eating something.

Maybe you gagged.

Maybe you choked.

Maybe someone forced you to eat something you hated.

Write that one down too.

Food:

Feeling:

Notice something?

The food isn't what stands out.

The feeling does.

Children are no different.

When Food Stops Feeling Safe

Today I understand that a child's first negative food experience can happen for many different reasons.

Maybe chewing was difficult.

Maybe the texture felt overwhelming.

Maybe their stomach hurt.

Maybe they gagged.

Maybe they had reflux.

Maybe they simply weren't developmentally ready for that food yet.

Those underlying reasons are important, and they are part of the larger Foodology framework.

But for this chapter, the reason isn't what matters most.

What matters is what the child's brain learns next.

Imagine little John is eighteen months old.

He takes a bite of a cooked carrot.

Maybe the piece was too large.

Maybe he couldn't move it to his molars.

Maybe it felt mushy and unpredictable.

Maybe he gagged.

Whatever the reason...

His brain reaches one conclusion.

"This doesn't feel safe."

The next time he sees that carrot, he's not making a logical decision.

He's remembering a feeling.

That's where mindset begins.

The Mismatch

Now let's look at the exact same moment through two different sets of eyes.

PARENT'S MINDSET	CHILD'S MINDSET
"These carrots are healthy."	*"That food didn't feel safe."*
"I want my child to grow."	*"I don't want to feel that again."*
"I know they liked them yesterday."	*"I'm trying to protect myself."*
"I just need one more bite."	

Neither person is wrong.

They're simply working from two completely different realities.

And that mismatch is where many mealtime battles begin.

Every Experience Adds Another Brick

Every experience we have with food leaves an impression.

Positive experiences build trust.

Negative experiences build hesitation.

Imagine every negative food experience as a single brick.

One brick isn't a problem.

But meal after meal...

Day after day...

Those bricks slowly become a wall.

Eventually that wall becomes what parents describe as "picky eating."

I see it differently.

I see a child protecting themselves based on the experiences they've had.

And here's the hopeful part...

If negative experiences can build the wall...

Positive experiences can slowly take it down.

That's why this book isn't about getting one more bite.

It's about creating one more positive experience.

Because regardless of whether the original challenge came from gut health, sensory processing, oral motor skills, or something else entirely, the mindset that develops afterward plays a powerful role in what happens next.

That's why we're starting here.

Key Takeaways

- Children aren't trying to be difficult—they're trying to communicate something they may not yet have the words to express.

- The first negative food experience can happen for many different reasons, but what matters next is the meaning your child attaches to that experience.

- Positive and negative food experiences build over time. Every meal is an opportunity to strengthen trust or add another brick to the wall.

- Lasting feeding progress begins when we stop asking, "How do I get my child to eat?" and start asking, "What is my child trying to communicate?"

- A child's relationship with food is built one experience at a time—and that relationship can be changed.

Action Steps

1. Complete the Food Memories Worksheet for yourself.

2. Complete the Negative Food Experiences Worksheet from your child's perspective. What experiences might have taught them that certain foods don't feel safe?

3. This week, notice every time your child communicates something about food. Before reacting, pause and ask yourself:

"What might my child be trying to tell me?"

CHAPTER THREE

Rewriting Success

*"If you don't redefine success, you'll spend
every meal feeling like you're failing."*

For years, I measured success the same way many parents and therapists still do today.

How many bites did they eat?

Did they lick the food?

Did they chew it?

Did they swallow it?

Did they finish their dinner?

Those were the victories I celebrated.

The problem?

Those measurements don't tell us whether a child is actually building a healthy relationship with food.

A child can comply.

A child can take five bites.

A child can even finish an entire meal...

...while becoming more anxious about eating every single day.

Compliance and confidence are not the same thing.

That realization completely changed the way I practice feeding therapy—and it might just change the way you approach dinner tonight.

The Wrong Scoreboard

Imagine you're coaching your child's soccer team.

Would you judge their entire season based on how many goals they scored during the very first game?

Of course not.

You'd celebrate showing up.

Trying.

Learning.

Passing.

Working as a team.

Building confidence.

Eating is no different.

Children don't become confident eaters overnight.

Confidence is built through hundreds of small, positive experiences.

Yet somehow, when it comes to feeding, we keep looking at the scoreboard.

"How many bites?"

"Did they eat the broccoli?"

"Did they finish?"

What if we've been keeping score all wrong?

A New Definition of Success

Let's rewrite the scoreboard.

Instead of measuring what your child ate, begin measuring how they experienced the meal.

Success might look like...

> Coming to the table without a fight.
>
> Helping prepare dinner.
>
> Looking at a new food.
>
> Tolerating a new food on their plate.
>
> Smelling a food they've always avoided.
>
> Touching it.
>
> Talking about it.
>
> Playing with it.
>
> Asking questions.
>
> Staying calm when a new food is served.
>
> Saying "No thank you" respectfully.
>
> Remaining engaged with the family, even if they don't eat the new food.

Read that list again.

Those are all signs of progress.

They may not feel exciting.

But they're exactly the kinds of moments that eventually lead to lasting change.

The Bites Will Come

One of the hardest truths for parents to accept is this:

You cannot rush confidence.

Trying to force the last step before the first steps are ready only creates more pressure.

It's like expecting a child to run before they've learned to crawl.

Every positive experience lays another brick in the foundation.

Every safe interaction with food tells your child's brain:

"Maybe this isn't so scary after all."

That's the progress we're looking for.

Because when confidence grows...
Curiosity follows.

When curiosity grows...
Trying follows.

When trying grows...
Eating follows.

Notice where eating appears?

At the end.

Not the beginning.

The Power of Your Focus

Have you ever noticed that once you're thinking about buying a certain car, you suddenly start seeing it everywhere?

That happened to me when I was looking at a Mazda.

Before I started researching it, I barely noticed them.

Then suddenly...

They were everywhere.

Did everyone on Long Island rush out and buy a Mazda overnight?

Of course not.

My brain simply decided that Mazdas were important, so it began noticing them.

This is one of the incredible jobs of your brain.

Every second of every day, you're surrounded by millions of pieces of information. Your brain has to decide what deserves your attention. The Reticular Activating System, often called the RAS, acts as a filter. It pays attention to the things you've taught it are important and quietly ignores thousands of others.

The same thing happens at your dinner table.

If your brain is constantly looking for evidence that...

> *"My child isn't eating."*
>
> *"They're being difficult."*
>
> *"Dinner is always a disaster."*
>
> *"They never make progress."*

...guess what you'll notice?

Exactly those things.

But what if we changed the target?

What if, instead, you trained your brain to notice progress?

Maybe your child stayed at the table two minutes longer.

Maybe they stirred the spaghetti sauce.

Maybe they tolerated broccoli on their plate without tears.

Maybe they smelled a new food.

Maybe they smiled during dinner.

Those moments matter.

In fact, they're often the very moments that eventually lead to bigger breakthroughs.

The more you train yourself to notice progress, the more progress you'll begin to see.

No, you're not pretending problems don't exist.

You're simply teaching your brain to recognize growth that was already happening.

And here's the beautiful part...

When parents begin noticing success...

Their children often begin feeling successful too.

That's where confidence begins.

And confidence changes everything.

Key Takeaways

- Success isn't measured by bites—it's measured by confidence.

- Compliance and confidence are not the same thing.

- Every positive mealtime experience lays another brick in your child's foundation.

- What you choose to measure shapes what you notice—and what you notice influences where you put your energy.

Action Steps

Redefine Success

For the next three dinners, don't count bites.

Instead, write down five successes from each meal.

Maybe your child:

- Came to the table without protesting.
- Stayed one minute longer than yesterday.
- Helped stir the spaghetti sauce.
- Tolerated a new food on their plate.
- Smelled a new food.
- Looked at a new food.
- Stayed calm.
- Laughed with the family.
- Asked a question about a food.

The goal isn't to pretend everything is perfect.

The goal is to train your brain to recognize the progress that was already happening.

At the end of three days, ask yourself:

> *"What successes would I have completely missed before reading this chapter?"*

CHAPTER FOUR

Knowing When to Push—and When to Pause

Matching the Challenge to Your Child

By now, you may be wondering something.

> *"Okay Christine… if pressure is so harmful, why does it seem to work?"*

It's a fair question.

Imagine telling your child,

> *"If you don't eat your carrots, there's no TV tonight."*

Your child sighs, picks up the carrot, takes a bite, and swallows it.

From the outside, that looks like success.

The carrot was eaten.

The behavior changed.

So why wouldn't we keep doing that?

For a long time, I believed that was exactly what success looked like.

Early in my career, I was trained primarily in behavioral approaches to feeding. I worked with children with autism and measured progress through observable behaviors. Children earned tokens for touching a food, licking it, tasting it, or taking a bite. We celebrated measurable progress because those were the tools I had been taught.

I wasn't trying to do anything harmful.

I was using the best information I had at the time.

And to be fair...

It often worked.

Children took more bites.

They completed the task.

The data looked great.

But over time, something didn't sit right with me.

Were these children becoming more comfortable with food...

...or were they simply becoming better at complying?

Later, after completing the SOS Approach to Feeding, I realized something I had completely misunderstood.

The Steps to Eating hierarchy was never meant to be a behavior chart.

It was meant to describe a child's natural journey toward feeling safe enough to explore food.

Instead of trying to move children up the hierarchy through rewards and compliance, the goal became creating enough positive sensory experiences that they wanted to move up the hierarchy themselves.

So I stopped asking,

> *"How do I get another bite?"*

Instead I began asking,

> *"How do I help this child feel safe enough to take the next step?"*

Which, by the way, was a harder question to answer. And it wasn't as neat and tidy as a behavioral chart was.

But compliance and confidence are not the same thing. Neither are compliance and curiosity, or compliance and enjoyment.

A person can comply with enough pressure. But they cannot be pressured into feeling safe. And safety is what allows confidence—and eventually enjoyment—to grow.

But Wait... Didn't My Parents Push Me?

At this point you might be thinking,

> *"My parents pushed me all the time."*

Maybe they made you stick with piano lessons.

Maybe they made you keep going to soccer practice.

Maybe they insisted you finish swimming lessons, even though you cried every week.

And maybe today you're grateful they did.

So...

Why should food be any different?

I've wrestled with that question myself.

One of the greatest lessons I've learned about feeding didn't happen at the dinner table.

It happened at the pool.

My son has always had an interesting relationship with water.

For a while, he hated getting water on his face (bath time was super fun for a while there!). Eventually, that became okay.

Then he didn't want water on his head.

Later, he tolerated that too.

Then came putting his face underwater.

Then jumping into the pool.

Every new step felt impossible...

...until it wasn't.

As a former swim instructor, I was probably more particular than most parents about where I enrolled him.

The first swim school was not my cup of tea.

The instructors were kind.

The kids laughed.

They splashed.

Everyone had fun.

My son loved going.

But by the end of the session...

He still couldn't really swim.

As much as I appreciated how warm the instructors were, I found myself thinking,

> *"We're keeping everyone comfortable... but we're never asking them to grow."*

So I enrolled him somewhere else.

This program was different.

The expectations were higher.

Some children cried during the first few lessons.

But I noticed something fascinating.

The instructors never started with the hardest thing.

They didn't walk children to the twelve-foot end on the first day.

They didn't dunk them underwater.

They didn't laugh at their fears or tell them to "just do it."

Instead, they built trust.

They held the children close.

They talked to them.

They made them laugh.

They distracted them with games.

Five minutes earlier, a child had been clinging to their parent in tears.

Now they were smiling, splashing, and forgetting they had been afraid.

Week after week, the challenges grew.

One day my son proudly put his face underwater for the first time.

We celebrated.

Not because he had mastered swimming...

But because he had mastered the next step.

A few weeks later, I watched the class walk toward the twelve-foot end of the pool.

I could hear my son negotiating with his instructor.

> *"Please don't make me."*

> *"I'm not ready."*

> *"I don't want to."*

There weren't just one or two instructors waiting.

There were three.

Every safety measure was in place.

The instructor gently encouraged him forward.

He protested.

He hesitated.

And then…

He jumped.

He went under for just a second before three waiting instructors helped him back up.

That experience taught me something I'll never forget.

Yes…

My son was challenged.

In fact, if you had asked him in that moment, he probably would have told you I was making him do something he wasn't ready for.

But here's the difference.

We didn't start there.

Before that jump, he had already spent weeks building trust.

Weeks learning that water could be fun.

Weeks putting his face in.

Weeks floating.

Weeks kicking.

Weeks succeeding.

The jump into the deep end wasn't Step One.

It was Step Thirty.

Imagine if we had started there on the very first day.

Can you picture it?

He probably would have wrapped himself around my leg. Refused to get into the pool. Maybe even refused to walk into the building the following week.

Because the challenge far exceeded his sense of safety.

That isn't how great swim instructors teach.

And it isn't how we should approach feeding.

Children don't grow because we eliminate every challenge. They also don't grow because we skipped over all the steps in between.

They grow because we carefully match the challenge to the confidence they've already built.

Feeding follows the same principle.

But in many ways, it's even more complex.

Water is always water.

Food changes.

Its temperature changes.

Its texture changes.

Its smell changes.

It changes as we chew it.

Then our bodies have to digest it.

Some children experience pain.

Some have sensory differences.

Some have oral motor challenges.

Some have all three.

And unlike swimming lessons, we don't practice once a week.

We practice eating several times every single day.

That's why matching the challenge to the child matters so much.

Not every child needs less challenge.

Not every child needs more challenge.

Every child needs the right challenge at the right time.

So... How Do You Know?

This is the question I want every parent to ask before every meal.

"Does my child need more safety today... or are they ready for a gentle challenge?"

Let's look at two very different children.

- Eats only one specific brand of chicken nuggets.
- Refuses a preferred food if it's cut differently.
- Notices tiny changes in packaging or presentation.
- Gags or panics around unfamiliar foods.
- Avoids touching new foods.
- Becomes distressed when foods are too close together.
- Has a very small number of safe foods.

This child isn't being stubborn. Their nervous system is telling us, "I don't feel safe yet."

Our job isn't to push harder. Our job is to build more safety.

- Accepts different brands without distress.
- Enjoys exploring foods.
- Tolerates different textures.
- Tries new foods willingly.
- Can recover after an uncomfortable bite.
- Eats a fairly wide variety but struggles to expand consistency or quantity.

This child already has a solid foundation.

Now they may benefit from gentle coaching and appropriately matched challenges.

Do you see the difference?

The food didn't determine the strategy.

The child did.

That's why there isn't one "right" feeding strategy.

The same challenge that helps one child grow may overwhelm another.

And the same strategy that overwhelms one child may be exactly what another child needs.

The goal isn't to memorize techniques.

The goal is to learn to read your child.

One of My Favorite Ways to Remove Pressure

One of my favorite ways to reduce pressure actually doesn't happen at the table.

It happens before the meal ever begins.

In the kitchen.

When children help prepare food, the goal is no longer eating.

The goal is helping.

Mixing.

Pouring.

Washing vegetables.

Measuring flour.

Stirring soup.

Setting the table.

Food becomes something you're working with, rather than something someone is waiting for you to eat.

Sometimes children naturally become more curious and may smell, lick, or taste ingredients along the way.

Sometimes they don't.

And that's okay.

That isn't the goal.

The goal is simply creating positive, pressure-free experiences with food outside of mealtime.

Those experiences matter.

Every interaction with food doesn't have to end with eating to be valuable.

Key Takeaways

- Compliance and confidence are not the same thing. A child can comply with enough pressure without ever feeling safe enough to enjoy food.

- Challenge isn't the enemy—poorly timed challenge is. Lasting growth happens when the challenge matches your child's current level of safety and confidence.

- Safety builds confidence, and confidence makes the next challenge possible. Just like my son didn't start in the twelve-foot end of the pool, our children shouldn't be expected to start at the hardest step with food.

- The best feeding strategy depends on the child in front of you. Learning to read your child's cues is more valuable than memorizing techniques.

Action Steps

4. Before each meal this week, pause and ask yourself:

"Does my child need more safety today... or are they ready for a gentle challenge?"

5. After the meal, write down one observation that helped you answer that question. Focus on your child's body language, emotions, and behavior rather than how many bites they took.

6. If you catch yourself wanting to push, pause and ask yourself:

"Am I asking my child to jump into the twelve-foot end... or are they truly ready for this next step?"

Change Your Home

Now we build the environment where lasting change can actually happen— our Mealtime Agreements.

CHAPTER FIVE

The Mealtime Agreements

Creating Safety Through Structure

___

Why We Call Them Agreements

You'll notice I don't call these Mealtime Rules.

I call them Mealtime Agreements.

Words matter.

Rules tell people what they can't do.

Agreements help everyone know what to expect.

Agreements feel different.

An agreement is something everyone understands and participates in.

It creates predictability.

And predictability creates safety.

Think about the last time you went to your favorite restaurant.

You probably didn't spend much time wondering what was going to happen next.

Someone greeted you.

You were shown to a table.

You were handed a menu.

The server gave you a few minutes to decide.

They came back to take your order.

Your food arrived.

You ate.

You paid.

Then you left.

There was never a moment where you wondered,

> *"Wait... what happens now?"*

Imagine if there weren't any structure.

The server asked for your order before giving you a menu.

Your entrée arrived before your drink.

Halfway through dinner someone asked you to move to another table.

The check showed up before your food.

You'd probably leave feeling frustrated—not because the food was bad, but because nothing made sense.

Restaurants work because everyone understands the rhythm. We've all collectively agreed upon a set of things that happen in a certain order. So if you go to Brazil, Japan, America, or Italy, they all function about the same.

Not because there are lots of rules.

Because there are shared expectations.

Children need that same predictability.

When they know what comes next, their nervous system can relax.

Instead of spending energy figuring out what's happening...

They can spend that energy learning.

That's exactly what our Mealtime Agreements are designed to do.

They're not rules.

They're the predictable rhythm that allows children—and parents—to feel safe enough to enjoy meals together.

Our Four Mealtime Agreements

These four agreements are the foundation of everything we do at Foodology.

Before we focus on expanding foods...

Before we work on taking bites...

Before we tackle picky eating...

We first create an environment where learning can actually happen.

These agreements are designed to reduce stress, increase predictability, and help everyone at the table know what to expect.

Don't worry if they feel overwhelming at first.

You don't need to master all four overnight.

In fact, in our coaching program we spend weeks helping families implement these one step at a time because we've learned something important:

Everything else builds on these agreements.

Think of them as the foundation of your home.

Without a strong foundation, every strategy you build on top of it becomes much harder to sustain.

Here are the four agreements we'll be learning together.

Mealtimes Happen at the Table

Our tables become a predictable place for eating, connecting, and learning—and our bodies stay there too, so the brain can focus on the meal. Predictability creates safety, and safety is the foundation for everything that follows.

Meals Have a Beginning and an End

Predictable routines create predictable nervous systems. We'll look at meal timing, snacks, grazing, transitions, and why knowing when a meal begins—and when it ends—helps children feel safe and learn the language of their own bodies.

Everyone Has a Job

Grown-ups decide what, when, and where food is offered. Children decide whether and how much to eat. One of the most powerful mindset shifts you'll make as a parent—it reduces power struggles while helping children reconnect with their own hunger, fullness, and confidence.

We Speak Respectfully About Food

The words we use shape the way children think and feel about food. We'll replace pressure, judgment, and negativity with language that builds curiosity and confidence.

Each of these agreements may seem simple.

But don't underestimate them.

Simple doesn't mean easy.

Families often tell us these agreements transformed their mealtimes long before their child started eating new foods.

Why?

Because children don't learn best in chaos.

They learn best in environments that feel safe, predictable, and connected.

And that's exactly what these agreements are designed to create.

. . .

Mealtimes Happen at the Table

PART ONE
Why This Agreement Matters

One of the very first agreements we establish with every family is simple:

Mealtimes happen at the table.

It sounds almost too simple to matter.

But I promise you...

This one agreement lays the foundation for everything that comes next.

Think about driving a car.

We all stop at red lights.

We drive on the correct side of the road.

We wait our turn at a four-way stop.

None of us particularly enjoy waiting at red lights, but we follow these agreements because they keep everyone safe and make life predictable.

Mealtimes work the same way.

Children shouldn't have to wonder…

"Where am I eating today?"

"Can I take my food into the living room?"

"Can I walk around while I eat?"

"Can I eat in front of the television?"

The decision has already been made.

Predictability creates safety.

And safety creates the best environment for learning.

Your "Table" Doesn't Have to Be a Table

When I say,

"Mealtimes happen at the table,"

I'm not talking about one specific piece of furniture.

Maybe your family eats at the kitchen table.

Maybe you gather in the dining room.

Maybe your home is small and everyone naturally eats around the coffee table.

That's perfectly okay.

The agreement isn't about owning a fancy dining room.

The agreement is about deciding where eating happens.

Whatever place your family chooses…

That's your table.

That's your family's mealtime space.

And once that place has been chosen…

That's where mealtimes happen.

A Restaurant You'd Never Forget

Imagine you're eating dinner at a nice restaurant.

Halfway through your meal, the family next to you stands up.

Dad walks toward the television in the bar carrying his steak.

Mom is wandering around talking on her phone while eating her salad.

One child runs laps through the restaurant with chicken nuggets in their hand.

Another bumps into your chair with spaghetti hanging out of their mouth.

Crumbs are everywhere.

Someone spills a drink.

People are weaving between the tables carrying plates of food.

Sounds ridiculous, doesn't it?

You'd probably wonder,

"What in the world is going on?"

Because we've all silently agreed that meals happen at the table.

It's simply part of how people eat together.

Our homes deserve that same predictability.

Now, I'll be honest.

Part of this agreement is practical.

Food scattered throughout the house creates crumbs, sticky furniture, extra cleaning, and sometimes even bugs or rodents.

But that's actually not my biggest concern.

My biggest concern is safety.

Children should never be walking, running, climbing, jumping, or playing with food in their mouths.

As a feeding therapist, I take choking risk very seriously.

When parents ask me how to explain this agreement to their child, I encourage them to simply tell the truth.

> *"Food stays at the table because it's the safest place for our bodies to eat."*

Children understand safety.

Just like we buckle seatbelts, wear helmets, and hold hands while crossing the street...

This is simply one of the ways we keep our bodies safe.

The decision has already been made.

Our Bodies Stay at the Table Too

This agreement isn't just about where the food stays.

It's also about where our bodies stay.

One of the most common challenges we see with picky eaters isn't simply refusing food.

It's wandering.

A child takes one bite...

Then gets up to pet the dog.

They come back.

Take another bite.

Then run to grab crayons.

Or they hop off the chair to jump around the room before returning for another bite.

Sometimes they never really sit at all.

They're kneeling.

Standing.

Leaning over the chair.

Eating while pacing around the room.

Parents often tell me,

> *"But they're still eating!"*

And that's true.

But every time your child's body leaves the table...

Their attention leaves the meal too.

Now their brain is focused on toys.

The dog.

The television.

The crayons.

The meal never truly becomes the focus.

One of our goals is helping your child's brain connect one simple idea:

When my body is at the table, it's time to eat.

That doesn't mean children need to sit perfectly still.

They're children.

They'll wiggle.

They'll shift.

Sometimes they'll need a quick bathroom break.

That's all normal.

But we don't want mealtime stretching across the entire house.

Meals have a place.

Food has a place.

And whenever possible...

Our bodies stay there too.

This Agreement Applies to Everyone

One mistake I see families make is expecting only the child to follow this agreement.

Meanwhile...

Mom is eating dinner standing at the kitchen counter.

Dad is eating on the couch watching television.

An older sibling grabs a snack and heads upstairs.

Children notice these things.

If we want our children to believe mealtimes happen together in one predictable place...

We have to model that too.

Now, I know real life is busy.

Parents work late.

Schedules don't always line up.

Perfection isn't the goal.

Connection is.

Whenever possible, choose one meal each day—or even a few meals each week—where everyone gathers in your family's mealtime space.

Because we're not just teaching children where to eat.

We're teaching them what family meals feel like.

Making It Work in Real Life

Whenever we introduce this agreement in our coaching program, I hear many of the same questions.

Let's walk through some of the biggest ones.

"My child only eats while watching TV."

You're not alone.

This is probably one of the most common concerns parents bring to us.

The important thing to remember is this:

Right now, we're changing where eating happens—not everything about how your child eats.

If television has been part of your family's mealtime routine for years, don't expect your child to happily sit at the table with no support on Day One.

Instead...

Bring the television to the table.

I know that might surprise you.

But remember...

We're changing one thing at a time.

If watching television has helped your child stay calm and regulated during meals, removing the television and changing where they eat at the same time is often too much change.

We'll gradually fade distractions later in the program.

For now, our goal is simple:

Mealtimes happen at the table.

As your child becomes more comfortable, consider transitioning from television to music.

Music is often easier to fade than a screen while still providing a familiar routine.

"My child won't even come to the table."

Again...

Very common.

Introducing a new agreement doesn't mean your child automatically has the skills to follow it.

Some children need transition warnings.

Some benefit from visual schedules.

Some respond well to visual timers that count down until mealtime.

If your child doesn't understand time yet, use meaningful events instead.

> *"After Bluey is over..."*

> *"After we pick up your sister..."*

> *"After we clean up your toys..."*

These kinds of cues help children predict what's coming next.

If your child is deeply engaged in play, allow them to bring one small toy to the table during the transition.

Think of it like bringing a security blanket into a new environment.

As mealtimes become more comfortable, you'll gradually fade that support.

"My child comes to the table… but won't stay there."

This is actually a different challenge.

Some children happily come to the table.

They just can't seem to stay.

One bite.

Up to pet the dog.

Back for another bite.

Off to grab crayons.

Back again.

Instead of seeing this as defiance, remember…

Sitting for a meal is a skill.

Calmly guide your child back to the table each time.

Over time, they'll begin staying a little longer.

Just like every other skill in this book…

We're building it gradually.

Comfort Matters More Than You Think

One of the biggest reasons children struggle to stay seated has nothing to do with behavior.

They're uncomfortable.

Imagine trying to eat dinner while sitting on a tall bar stool with your feet dangling in the air.

How long would it take before you started shifting, swinging your legs, or standing up?

Children are no different.

Their hips, knees, and feet should all be well supported.

When the body feels stable, the nervous system feels safer.

And when the nervous system feels safer...

The brain can focus on eating.

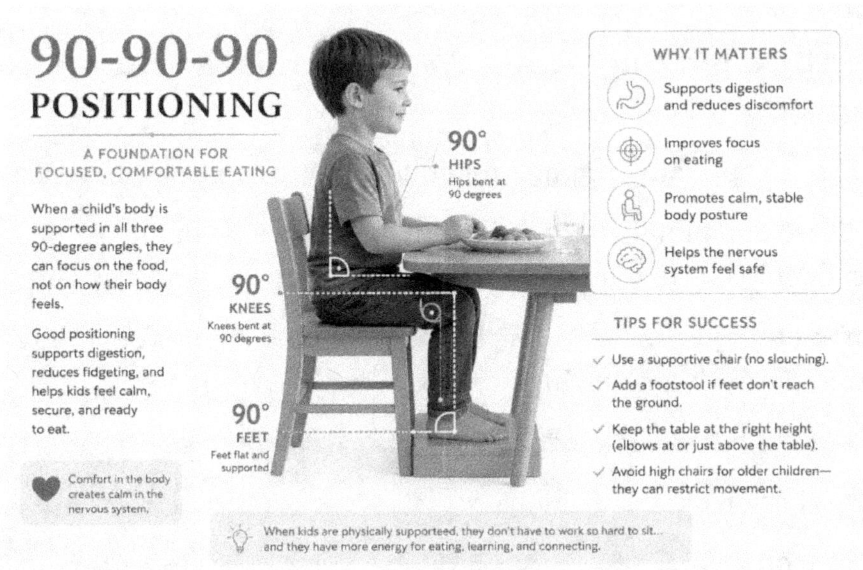

"We don't all eat together."

That's okay.

Life happens.

Parents work different shifts.

Children have activities.

The goal isn't perfection.

The goal is creating as many opportunities for connection as your family's schedule allows.

Even one consistent family meal each day—or a few each week—is a wonderful place to start.

If everyone can't eat together...

That's okay.

The agreement still stays the same.

Mealtimes happen at the table.

"My child can't stand the smell or look of our food."

This is especially common for children with sensory differences.

Please don't interpret this agreement to mean your child suddenly has to tolerate every smell or every food on Day One.

If another person's meal feels overwhelming, invite your child into the problem-solving process.

"What could we do to make this feel a little easier?"

Maybe you open a window.

Turn on a fan.

Move seats.

Sit farther away.

These are temporary accommodations while your child's nervous system learns that the table is a safe place to be.

Introducing the Agreement

If your family has always eaten in different rooms, expect this to feel a little awkward at first.

You're changing a family culture.

That takes time.

Your child may ask,

> *"Can I eat on the couch?"*

> *"Can I take this into the living room?"*

> *"Can I just watch one more show?"*

Instead of debating...

Simply remind them of the agreement.

> *"Remember, mealtimes happen at the table because it's the safest place for our bodies to eat."*

Keep it short.

Keep it calm.

Keep it predictable.

The decision has already been made.

Will there be exceptions?

Absolutely.

Movie nights.

Road trips.

Picnics.

Special celebrations.

Life isn't rigid.

But while you're building this new habit, consistency is your friend.

Children learn what to expect by experiencing the same expectation over and over again.

That's how agreements become routines.

Routines become habits.

And habits become family culture.

Key Takeaways

- Mealtimes happen in one predictable place.
- Food stays at the table because it's the safest place to eat.
- Our bodies stay at the table so our brains can focus on the meal.
- Comfort matters. Proper seating and foot support help children stay engaged.
- Parents model mealtime agreements too.
- Consistency—not perfection—is what builds family routines.

Action Steps

7. Decide where your family's mealtime space will be.

8. Introduce the agreement using one simple sentence:

"Mealtimes happen at the table because it's the safest place for our bodies to eat."

9. Practice eating in that same space this week whenever possible.

10. If your child gets up during the meal, calmly guide them back without arguing or lecturing.

11. Look at your child's seating. Are their hips, knees, and feet supported? If not, make one adjustment before your next meal.

12. If your child asks to eat somewhere else, calmly repeat the agreement rather than negotiating.

13. Before your next meal, look around your mealtime space and ask yourself:

"Does this space communicate that mealtimes matter?"

Clear away clutter if needed and create a place where your family can gather—not just to eat, but to connect.

. . .

Meals Have a Beginning and an End

PART ONE
Why This Agreement Matters

Let me paint a picture.

It's 10:00 in the morning.

Your child grabs two Cheerios from a bowl sitting on the counter.

Then they're off to play.

Five minutes later they wander back for one bite of toast.

Then they're building with Legos.

A few minutes later, you find yourself following them through the house with a spoon.

"Just one more bite!"

They take a bite while running down the hallway.

Then they're gone again.

Sound familiar?

If you're like many of the families we work with, you might be thinking,

"Well… at least they're eating something."

I understand why parents do this.

When you're worried your child isn't eating enough, one more bite feels like a victory.

But here's the problem.

Your child didn't really eat a meal.

They took tiny bites scattered throughout their morning while their brain stayed focused on playing.

Eating became something happening in the background instead of becoming the main event.

Over time, meals become blurry.

Children stop learning:

"Now we're eating."

and

"Now we're finished eating."

Instead, food is available all day long.

This is what we call *grazing*.

And while it almost always comes from a place of love, it accidentally creates another problem.

Your child never has the opportunity to become hungry.

Hunger Is a Good Thing

I know that sentence might make you a little uncomfortable.

As parents, we spend so much of our lives trying to prevent our children from feeling hungry that we've forgotten something important.

Hunger isn't dangerous.

It's information.

It's one of the body's most important ways of communicating.

Just like your body tells you when you're tired...

Or thirsty...

Or too hot...

Or need to use the bathroom...

It also tells you when it needs fuel.

When food is available every few minutes, your child's body never has the opportunity to send that message.

We're not trying to create hunger.

We're protecting your child's opportunity to experience it naturally.

Because children don't learn hunger because we talk about hunger.

They learn hunger by experiencing it.

And when children begin to experience predictable hunger before meals, they often become much more interested in eating.

But there's an even bigger reason this agreement matters.

Learning the Language of the Body

A few months ago, one of the families in our program made a discovery that completely changed the way they understood their son.

Every night before bed, he became anxious.

He paced.

He couldn't settle.

He became emotional.

His parents assumed he had bedtime anxiety.

After all, it happened almost every night.

Then one evening they offered him a small bedtime snack.

Within minutes...

The anxiety disappeared.

He calmly got ready for bed.

No tears.

No pacing.

No struggle.

Another thing they noticed?

Sometimes during the day he would simply stare off into space.

Again, they assumed he was distracted.

It turned out that was another one of his body's clues.

He wasn't anxious.

He wasn't distracted.

He was hungry.

His body had been communicating all along.

He just hadn't learned its language yet.

What my client's parents had discovered was something called *interoception.*

> **INTEROCEPTION**
> Our ability to notice and understand what's happening inside our bodies.

It's how we recognize things like:

> *"I'm thirsty."*
>
> *"I'm tired."*
>
> *"I'm too hot."*
>
> *"My tummy feels empty."*
>
> *"My stomach feels full."*

For some children, these signals are obvious.

For others, they're confusing—or they don't recognize them at all.

Many children experience hunger differently.

Some become silly.

Some become emotional.

Some become quiet.

Some become anxious.

Some become irritable.

Some lose focus.

Some become extra clingy.

The goal isn't simply to get children to eat.

The goal is to help them recognize what their own bodies are trying to tell them.

And this is where grazing becomes such a problem.

When children nibble throughout the day, they rarely experience the natural rhythm of hunger and fullness.

Their body never has the opportunity to clearly communicate,

> *"I'm hungry."*

Then…

> *"I'm comfortably full."*

Children don't learn hunger because we explain hunger.

They learn hunger by experiencing it.

Predictable meals and snacks give children hundreds of opportunities to practice recognizing those internal signals.

And over time…

Those signals become easier to recognize.

PART TWO

Putting This Agreement Into Practice

Whenever we introduce this agreement in our coaching program, parents usually ask many of the same questions.

Let's walk through them together.

"How often should my child eat?"

One of the first questions parents ask is,

"Okay... so how often should I actually offer food?"

In our practice, we typically recommend offering young children an opportunity to eat about every 2–3 hours throughout the day.

For most families, that naturally looks like three meals and two to three snacks.

For example:

> 8:00 AM — Breakfast
>
> 10:00 AM — Snack
>
> 12:00 PM — Lunch
>
> 3:00 PM — Snack
>
> 5:30 PM — Dinner
>
> 7:30 PM — Optional bedtime snack (depending on your child's age and nutritional needs)

Don't get hung up on the exact times.

The clock isn't the goal.

Predictability is.

Your child begins learning,

> *"There will always be another opportunity to eat."*

That predictability reduces anxiety around food while still allowing enough time for hunger to naturally develop between meals and snacks.

"But what if they're hungry?"

Good.

Not starving.

Hungry.

There's a difference.

Feeling hungry before a meal is exactly what we hope will happen.

It means your child's body is beginning to recognize its natural rhythm.

Many parents tell us,

> *"But they keep saying they're starving!"*

Take a deep breath.

Children are still learning the language of their bodies.

They may say they're starving when they're simply experiencing ordinary hunger.

That doesn't mean they're starving.

It means they're learning.

"My child asks for food fifteen minutes after the meal ends."

This is incredibly common.

Before ending the meal, give your child a gentle warning.

> *"Just so you know, once we leave the table, lunch will be all done until snack time."*

Then follow through.

If they ask for food fifteen minutes later, calmly remind them when the next opportunity to eat will be.

Instead of saying,

> *"No."*

Try saying,

> *"Lunch is all finished. We'll have snack after we pick up your sister."*

Or...

> *"We'll have snack after Bluey."*

Or...

> *"When this timer is all done."*

Young children don't understand clocks.

They understand routines.

Using another event in their day—or a visual timer that counts down—helps them understand when food will be available again.

Notice something important.

You aren't denying food.

You're teaching predictability.

"What if they have a meltdown?"

They might.

You're changing a family rhythm.

Change is hard.

Validate the feeling without changing the agreement.

> *"I know you're hungry."*

> *"Waiting is hard."*

> *"We'll have snack after bath time."*

Or...

"Dinner is after Daddy gets home."

You can comfort your child while still holding the boundary.

Consistency is what teaches predictability.

Predictability helps children feel safe.

"What if they just help themselves?"

One of our moms texted me one afternoon.

> *"Christine! We were trying the new schedule and my son walked into the pantry, opened the sugar container, and started eating it with a spoon!"*

Believe it or not…

That isn't unusual.

If your child truly cannot resist helping themselves to food yet, then the environment needs to support this new agreement.

That might mean:

Moving snacks out of reach.

Locking the pantry for a period of time.

Keeping preferred foods where only an adult can access them.

This isn't punishment.

It's support.

Think about it this way.

Imagine you've decided that bedtime is 8:00 every night.

If your child can simply turn the television back on, grab another toy, or decide bedtime doesn't apply to them…

Then bedtime isn't really a routine.

It's a suggestion.

The same is true for meals.

If food is always available whenever your child wants it, then meals don't really have a beginning and an end.

As your child develops this new rhythm, these supports can gradually fade.

"What about drinks?"

Many parents don't realize that grazing happens with drinks too.

Milk.

Juice.

Smoothies.

Even constantly sipping calorie-containing drinks throughout the day can reduce appetite because little tummies stay physically full.

Water is different.

Water should always be available.

But whenever possible, milk, juice, smoothies, and other calorie-containing beverages are best offered with meals and snacks.

This gives your child's appetite the opportunity to naturally build between eating opportunities.

"What if my child only eats three bites?"

Take a deep breath.

We're going to spend an entire chapter talking about that very question.

For now, remember this:

Your job is to provide predictable opportunities to eat.

Your child's job is deciding whether and how much to eat.

We'll build on that agreement in the next chapter.

But They Keep Asking…

One of the hardest parts of creating structured mealtimes isn't the schedule.

It's saying "not right now."

Many parents worry that setting limits around food means they're being mean or depriving their child.

It feels uncomfortable to hear,

> *"I'm hungry!"*

or

> *"Can I have crackers?"*

or

> *"I want ice cream!"*

So parents often give in—not because they believe it's the best choice, but because they don't want their child to feel disappointed.

Here's a simple mindset shift that can make this much easier.

Instead of thinking "no," think "later."

Those are two very different messages.

"No" feels final.

"Later" acknowledges your child's request while still protecting the routine you're trying to build.

> Instead of *"No, you can't have crackers."*
> Try *"Crackers aren't on the menu right now. We'll have another chance to eat after lunch."*
>
> Instead of *"No ice cream."*
> Try *"Ice cream isn't on today's menu. We can always plan for that another day."*

Or if your child doesn't yet understand the clock, use events instead of times.

> Instead of *"You can eat at 3:00."*
> Try *"After TV time."*
> *"After your sister gets home."*
> *"After we finish playing outside."*

Children understand routines much better than numbers on a clock.

Visual timers can also be incredibly helpful. Watching time count down or a color gradually change gives children something concrete to understand instead of simply hearing, "Wait."

Remember...

The goal isn't to deny food.

The goal is to create a predictable rhythm where your child's body has a chance to recognize hunger before the next eating opportunity arrives.

You're not saying,

> *"You can never have that."*

You're saying,

> *"Not this moment."*

And that's an important life skill.

One day your child will have to wait for dinner reservations, birthday cake, the popcorn at the movie theater, or lunch at school.

Learning that it's okay to wait doesn't create food anxiety.

When done with warmth and predictability, it actually builds flexibility, patience, and trust.

Your child learns something incredibly valuable:

> *"Just because I can't have it right now doesn't mean I'll never have it."*

That's a lesson that extends far beyond food.

Become an Interoception Detective

This week, don't count bites. Count observations.

Start paying attention to your child's body. What does hunger look like for your child? Do they become...

Quiet? Silly? Emotional? Anxious? Irritable? Distracted? Spacey? Extra clingy?

Remember our little friend from earlier? His "bedtime anxiety" turned out to be hunger. His body was communicating—he just hadn't learned its language yet.

Instead of immediately saying, "You're hungry," become curious. Try asking:

"What is your body telling you?"

"What does your tummy feel like?"

"Does your tummy feel empty, full, or somewhere in between?"

Help your child begin connecting body sensations with what they mean. Over time, they'll start recognizing these signals on their own—a skill they'll use for the rest of their life.

Key Takeaways

- Meals have a beginning and an end.

- Most young children do best with predictable opportunities to eat every 2–3 hours throughout the day.

- Grazing makes it harder for children to experience hunger and learn what hunger feels like.

- Hunger isn't something to fear—it's one of the body's most important ways of communicating.

- Predictable meal and snack times help children build healthy eating rhythms.

- Your job isn't to create hunger. Your job is to protect your child's opportunity to experience it naturally.

- Every child experiences hunger differently. Become curious about your child's unique body signals.

Action Steps

14. Create a simple meal and snack schedule that works for your family.

15. Before each meal ends, give your child a gentle warning:

"Once we're all done, we'll eat again at snack time."

16. If your child asks for food between meals, calmly tell them when the next opportunity to eat will be using another event in their day ("after school," "after bath," "after we pick up your sister") or a visual timer.

17. If your child is helping themselves to food between meals, adjust the environment so it supports your new agreement.

18. This week, become an Interoception Detective. Write down three ways your child communicates hunger besides saying, "I'm hungry."

Everyone Has a Job

PART ONE
Why This Agreement Matters

Imagine you've just finished making breakfast.

Maybe it's yogurt with fruit and toast.

You call your child to the table.

They sit down, look at the plate, and immediately say,

> *"I don't want this."*

> *"I want brownies."*

Or...

> *"I want chicken nuggets."*

Or...

> *"I want chocolate cereal."*

Sound familiar?

I had a little client named Adam who did exactly this.

His mom lovingly made him breakfast every morning.

She would put the plate in front of him.

He would look at it and say,

> *"No thanks. I want brownies."*

Wanting him to eat, she would head right back into the kitchen and make something different.

If he didn't want that...

She made something else.

Before she knew it, breakfast had become a restaurant where one very tiny customer got to rewrite the menu every five minutes.

I know exactly why she did it.

She wasn't trying to spoil him.

She wasn't weak.

She was trying to be a good mom.

She was worried he wouldn't eat.

And every parent reading this has probably done something similar.

There is absolutely no judgment here.

But over time, something interesting happens.

Children begin learning,

> *"If I wait long enough... something better will come."*

Without realizing it, we've accidentally taught them that the menu is negotiable.

That's exhausting for parents.

And it doesn't actually help children feel more secure around food.

Everyone Has a Job

One of the most influential feeding professionals in our field, Ellyn Satter, developed what she calls the Division of Responsibility in Feeding. Her work has shaped the way many feeding therapists—including me—think about mealtimes. Over the years, I've adapted those principles into the broader Foodology framework that we use with families every day.

Here's how I teach it.

Everyone has a job.

THE PARENT'S JOB	THE CHILD'S JOB
What food is offered.	Whether to eat.
When meals happen.	How much to eat.
Where meals happen.	

Notice what isn't on your child's list.

Choosing a completely different dinner after the meal has already been prepared.

And notice what isn't on the parent's list.

Deciding how many bites go into a child's mouth.

When everyone stays in their own lane…

Mealtimes become calmer.

The Safe Food Rule

Now…

This is where this advice often gets misunderstood.

Some people hear,

"Don't be a short-order cook."

And they think it means,

> *"Serve whatever you're eating. If your child doesn't like it, that's their problem."*

That isn't what I'm saying.

Remember what we've already learned.

We don't throw children into the deep end.

We match the challenge to the child.

At Foodology, we have one simple rule.

THE SAFE FOOD RULE

Every meal should include at least one safe food.

A safe food is something your child already knows how to eat comfortably.

Let's say you're making chicken curry for dinner.

You already know your child isn't ready for chicken curry.

That doesn't mean you make chicken nuggets.

Instead, maybe you also serve bread.

Apple slices.

Cheese.

Now your child has something familiar on the table.

Think about the last time you traveled somewhere unfamiliar.

Imagine walking into a restaurant where every single item on the menu is written in another language.

Nothing looks familiar.

Then suddenly...

You notice bread.

Instant relief.

You may not order your favorite meal.

But you know you won't leave hungry.

That's exactly what a safe food does.

It gives your child confidence to stay at the table without requiring you to make an entirely different meal.

Trusting Your Child's Body

This agreement isn't really about dinner.

It's about trust.

Trusting your child's body.

Years ago, my mom told me a story I'll never forget.

She was dating my dad and went to my grandparents' house for dinner.

She politely said she was full.

My grandfather encouraged her to eat more.

She declined again.

He kept insisting.

Eventually she felt too uncomfortable to keep saying no.

So she ate.

On the drive home...

She became so sick she had to pull over on the side of the road.

Think about that for a moment.

This wasn't a toddler.

This wasn't a picky eater.

This was a grown woman who ignored what her own body was telling her because someone else told her to keep eating.

How many times do we accidentally ask children to do the exact same thing?

> *"One more bite."*

> *"You barely ate."*

> *"You're not full."*

> *"Finish your plate."*

When we consistently override a child's internal body signals, we're teaching them to trust us more than they trust themselves.

I don't want that.

I want children to grow into adults who know how to listen to their bodies.

Sometimes Their Body Really Does Feel Full

We've worked with children who took only two or three bites of food before saying,

> *"I'm full."*

Parents often respond,

> *"There's no way you're full."*

And honestly…

I understand why.

From the outside, it doesn't seem possible.

But then we ran their gut microbiome testing.

Many had significant bloating.

Excess gas.

Constipation.

Their stomach really did feel full.

Their body wasn't lying.

It was communicating.

Imagine trying to pour more water into a sink that's already clogged.

There's nowhere for it to go.

The same thing can happen when a child is constipated.

If they haven't had a bowel movement in several days, eating may genuinely feel uncomfortable.

This is one of the reasons gut health is one of the four pillars of the Foodology Method.

Sometimes what looks like behavior is actually biology.

Trust the Process

I'll be honest with you.

This agreement is one of the hardest for parents to follow.

Not because it's difficult to understand.

Because it's difficult emotionally.

There's a voice inside almost every parent that says,

That thought doesn't make you a bad parent.

It makes you a loving one.

Every good parent wants their child to eat.

That's exactly why we have our Safe Food Rule.

Every meal includes at least one food your child already knows how to eat.

Notice...

I didn't say their favorite food.

I didn't say the meal has to be exactly what they wanted.

I simply said there should always be something on the plate they can comfortably eat.

That changes everything.

Now, if your child chooses not to eat...

It isn't because there was nothing they could eat.

It's because they're choosing not to eat what's being offered today.

That's different.

Think about going to a party.

Maybe none of the food is your favorite.

Maybe there's no pizza.

No tacos.

No sushi.

But you find something.

Maybe you eat the bread.

Maybe the fruit.

Maybe the cheese and crackers.

You make do until the next meal.

You don't panic.

You don't demand the host make you something different.

You adapt.

That's flexibility.

And that's exactly what we're teaching our children.

They are learning,

> *"My favorite food won't always be available, and that's okay."*

Because they also know something else.

Another opportunity to eat is coming.

Don't Accidentally Reward Skipping Meals

There's one place I see parents accidentally undermine this agreement.

Dinner is served.

Your child has a safe food on their plate.

They decide not to eat.

An hour later it's snack time.

They smile and say,

> *"I'll have ice cream!"*

If we immediately serve ice cream...

What did they just learn?

They learned they don't actually have to participate in dinner.

They simply have to wait for something better.

Without meaning to, we've turned snack time into the reward for skipping the meal.

That isn't the lesson we want to teach.

Instead, keep the next meal or snack consistent with your family's usual routine.

Another balanced eating opportunity.

Not a rescue meal.

Not a reward.

Remember…

We're teaching rhythm.

We're teaching flexibility.

We're teaching children that every meal won't be their favorite, and that's okay.

There will always be another opportunity to eat.

Key Takeaways

- Parents and children each have an important job at mealtimes.

- Parents decide what, when, and where food is offered.

- Children decide whether and how much they eat.

- Every meal should include at least one safe food.

- You are not a short-order cook, but you are a thoughtful meal planner.

- Sometimes what looks like behavior is actually biology. Gut health, constipation, bloating, and discomfort all influence appetite.

- Trusting your child's body helps them learn to trust it too.

- Flexibility grows when children know another opportunity to eat is always coming.

Action Steps

19. Write down your job and your child's job. Put
    the list on your refrigerator this week as a
    reminder.

20. Plan each meal with at least one safe food your
    child already eats comfortably.

21. If your child asks for something different after
    the meal has been served, calmly respond:

*"This is what's on the menu tonight. You don't have
to eat it, but this is what we're having."*

22. If your child says they're full, pause before
    responding. Instead of trying to convince them
    otherwise, become curious. Could their body be
    trying to tell you something?

23. Notice your own feelings this week. If your
    child doesn't eat, what comes up for you? Fear?
    Guilt? Frustration? Simply noticing your
    reaction is the first step toward changing it.

We Speak Respectfully About Food

PART ONE
Why This Agreement Matters

Imagine I walked into your kitchen carrying a dinner plate.

I smiled.

Set it in front of you.

Lifted the lid…

And underneath was a giant spider.

Would you eat it?

Probably not.

You'd probably say,

"Ew!"

"Gross!"

"No way!"

"Absolutely not!"

Now imagine I said,

"Just try one bite."

Still no?

Okay...

What if I told you it was packed with protein?

That it was incredibly healthy?

That people all over the world eat them?

Still no?

What if the chef came out and told you he'd spent three days preparing it?

Would that change your mind?

Probably not.

Why?

Because long before that spider ever reached your mouth...

Your brain had already made a decision.

"That isn't food."

Once our brains attach a strong emotion to something, convincing rarely works.

Our children do the exact same thing.

Long before food reaches their mouth, their brain often decides:

"Ew."

"Gross."

"Yuck."

"I don't eat that."

"That's Mommy's food."

Those words may seem harmless.

Every time a child says,

> *"I don't eat vegetables."*

Their brain hears,

> *"I'm someone who doesn't eat vegetables."*

Every time they say,

> *"That's gross."*

Their brain reinforces the idea that the food is something to avoid.

Before we can change eating...

We have to change the conversation.

Respecting Food Means Respecting People

One of our family agreements is simple.

We speak respectfully about food.

That doesn't mean you have to like every food.

It doesn't mean you have to eat every food.

It simply means we don't insult food—or the people who enjoy it.

Imagine you're eating a piece of fish for dinner.

Your child wrinkles their nose and shouts,

> *"EWWWW! THAT'S DISGUSTING!"*

Or...

"That smells so gross!"

Now imagine Grandma spent all afternoon making that meal.

Or you're at a friend's house.

Or in another country where that food is a family tradition.

Food is more than nutrition.

Food is culture.
Food is love.
Food is tradition.
Food is family.

We don't have to enjoy every food.

But we can always speak respectfully about it.

Instead of saying,

"That's disgusting."

We teach children to say,

"No thank you."

Or...

"I'm still learning about that food."

Or...

"That isn't my favorite."

Notice the difference.

One judges the food.

The other simply communicates a preference.

That's a life skill that extends far beyond your kitchen table.

We Describe Food Instead of Judging It

So what do we say instead?

We become food scientists.

Scientists don't say,

"Gross."

Scientists observe.

Instead of saying,

"It's yucky."

We ask,

"Tell me about it."

Help your child describe what they're noticing.

Is it...

    Hot or cold?
    Wet or dry?
    Smooth or bumpy?
    Crunchy or soft?
    Sweet or sour?
    Red or green?

Even smells can be described objectively.

Instead of,

"That smells disgusting!"

Try,

"That smell is really strong."

Or...

"That smell is really big."

Those are observations.

Not judgments.

And observations give us something to work with.

Imagine your child says,

> *"The strawberry is gross!"*

Instead, you help them discover,

> *"The strawberry feels wet."*

Now we have information.

Wet is something we can problem solve.

You might say,

> *"I wonder what would happen if we dried it with a paper towel."*

Or...

> *"Would it feel different if we held it with a fork?"*

We can't solve, "Gross."

But we can solve, "Wet."

One is an opinion.

The other is information.

Learning Is a Process

One of the biggest mindset shifts we teach in our program is this:

Learning takes time.

Children often believe that one bite is enough to make a lifelong decision.

"I tried it."

"I don't like it."

Case closed.

But that's not how learning works.

Think about riding a bike.

Reading.

Swimming.

Playing the piano.

No one expects to master those skills in one day.

Food works the same way.

Every time your child interacts with a food, their brain is collecting information.

How does it look?

How does it smell?

How does it feel?

How does it sound when I bite it?

How does it taste today?

One bite doesn't tell the whole story.

That's why one of our favorite words is...

Yet.

When your child says,

"I don't like it."

Simply respond,

> *"You don't like it... yet."*

We're still learning about it.

That tiny word changes everything.

Instead of becoming someone who doesn't eat strawberries...

Your child becomes someone who is still learning about strawberries.

Even when a child says,

> *"I LOVE IT!"*

I still respond the same way.

> *"You liked it today! We're still learning about it."*

Because food changes.

Recipes change.

Our bodies change.

Our preferences change.

Learning never really ends.

We aren't deciding forever today.

We're simply learning today.

PART TWO

Putting This Agreement Into Practice

This agreement takes practice.

At first, you'll probably feel like a broken record.

Your child says,

"Gross."

You say,

"Tell me about it."

They say,

"It's yucky."

You respond,

"What does it feel like?"

Over time, something incredible begins to happen.

Children start using this language on their own.

Instead of,

"Ew!"

They'll say,

"It's squishy."

Instead of,

"It smells gross."

They'll say,

"That smell is really strong."

Instead of,

"I don't eat that."

They'll begin saying,

"I'm still learning about that."

This isn't just changing words.

It's changing the way your child thinks.

Curiosity begins replacing judgment.

And curiosity is what opens the door to trying new foods.

Model the Language You Want to Hear

Children learn far more from what we model than what we correct. Listen to the way you talk about food.

Instead of *"I hate mushrooms."*

Try *"Mushrooms have a really earthy flavor."*

Instead of *"That smells terrible."*

Try *"That's a really strong smell."*

Your child is always listening. If we want respectful language from them, it starts with us.

Key Takeaways

- We speak respectfully about food—even foods we choose not to eat.

- Words shape beliefs, and beliefs shape identity.

- Describing food keeps curiosity alive. Judging food shuts curiosity down.

- Every food can be described using the five senses.

- We can't solve "gross," but we can solve "wet," "cold," "strong," or "bumpy."

- Learning about food is a process, not a one-time event.

- "Yet" reminds children that they are still learning.

Action Steps

24. Whenever your child says "ew," "gross," or "yuck," gently ask:

"Can you describe it instead?"

25. Practice using the five senses during one meal each day.

26. Introduce the word "yet." Every time your child says "I don't like it," respond with:

"You don't like it... yet. You're still learning about it."

27. Pay attention to your own language this week. Replace emotional words like "gross" or "disgusting" with objective descriptions.

28. Celebrate curiosity instead of conclusions. The goal isn't deciding whether a food is good or bad. The goal is learning something new about it.

PART III

Change Yourself

The most powerful tool in your child's feeding journey isn't a technique—it's you.

CHAPTER TEN

Why Are We Talking About You?

If you've made it this far, you may be wondering something.

"I bought this book because my child is the picky eater."

"Why are we suddenly talking about me?"

It's a fair question.

After all...

You're probably not the one refusing broccoli.

You're not hiding peas under your napkin.

You're not gagging when someone serves chicken.

So why would a feeding therapist spend an entire section talking about the parent?

Because children don't learn to eat in isolation.

They learn inside relationships.

And one of the biggest influences on your child's feeding journey...

...is you.

Before you panic...

This is not a chapter about blame.

It's a chapter about possibility.

Everything you've done up until this point has come from one place.

Love.

You begged because you were worried.

You bribed because you were desperate.

You made a second dinner because you didn't want your child to go hungry.

You chased your child around the house with a spoon because you thought one more bite might make the difference.

Not because you were a bad parent.

Because you were trying to be a good one.

Every decision you've made has been based on the information you had at the time.

Now you have new information.

And with new information comes new opportunities.

Is This Program for Everyone?

I'm going to tell you something that surprises a lot of people.

When parents call to learn more about our Unlocking Mealtimes program, my wonderful admin, Jackie, doesn't try to convince everyone to enroll.

In fact...

Sometimes she'll gently tell families that our program probably isn't the right fit.

That might sound like terrible business advice.

Wouldn't we want everyone to join?

Actually...

No.

Because not everyone is looking for the same thing.

Some parents are hoping someone else will fix the problem.

They imagine dropping their child off with a therapist, grabbing a coffee, scrolling on their phone for an hour, and coming back to a child who suddenly eats everything.

If only it worked that way.

Years ago, that's actually how we practiced.

Parents stayed in the waiting room.

We worked with the child.

At the end of the session we'd explain what we practiced and send everyone home.

The following week...

Very little had changed.

Not because the child wasn't capable.

Because nothing had changed during the other 167 hours of the week.

The therapist was working hard.

The child was working hard.

But home stayed exactly the same.

Progress was slow.

So we completely changed our model.

Parents came into the room.

They watched.

They practiced.

They asked questions.

They learned exactly what to say.

Exactly what not to say.

They became part of the therapy.

Everything changed.

Progress accelerated.

Not because we suddenly became better therapists.

Because therapy wasn't happening for one hour each week anymore.

It was happening every single day at home.

That's where lasting change happens.

The Greatest Surprise

After working with hundreds of families over the years, I've noticed something remarkable.

The biggest surprise isn't the foods children begin eating.

It isn't the calmer dinners.

It isn't even the progress we see in the child.

The biggest surprise...

Is the parent.

The parent who begins our program is rarely the same parent who finishes it.

Many parents come to us anxious.

They worry constantly.

They dread mealtimes before they even begin.

They second-guess every decision they make.

Many have loose boundaries because they're exhausted.

They've spent years negotiating.

Pleading.

Making separate meals.

Walking on eggshells.

Trying anything just to get one more bite.

Then...

Something starts to shift.

Not overnight.

But little by little.

They become calmer.

More confident.

They stop second-guessing themselves.

They know what to say.

Just as importantly...

They know what not to say.

Instead of reacting emotionally...

They begin responding intentionally.

Instead of asking,

> *"Why is my child doing this to me?"*

They begin asking,

> *"What is my child trying to communicate?"*

That one question changes everything.

They stop fighting their child…

And start understanding them.

Really understanding them.

The relationship around food improves.

But something even more important happens.

The relationship with their child improves.

Parents tell me all the time,

> *"I actually enjoy spending time with my child again."*
>
> *"I finally understand them."*
>
> *"I feel confident."*
>
> *"I'm not anxious anymore."*

The confidence they build around feeding doesn't stay at the dinner table.

It spills into every part of parenting.

And watching that transformation…

Honestly…

It's one of my favorite parts of my job.

Your Child May Be Your Greatest Teacher

There's something I've come to believe after all these years.

Our children are often our greatest teachers.

As much as we want to teach them…

They have an incredible way of teaching us.

Patience.

Flexibility.

Trust.

Presence.

Resilience.

And sometimes...

The very challenge you're facing today is carrying a lesson that you haven't discovered yet.

I know that can be hard to hear when you're exhausted.

When you're worried.

When every meal feels like a battle.

But I've watched it happen over and over again.

Parents begin the journey hoping their child will change.

Then somewhere along the way...

They realize they have changed too.

And once that happens...

Everything feels different.

Why This Matters

The next several chapters are going to challenge you.

Not your child.

You.

Some of the exercises will feel simple.

Others may stretch you.

Some might even make you uncomfortable.

Good.

Growth usually lives just outside our comfort zone.

Please don't skip them.

The parents who experience the biggest transformations aren't always the ones whose children have the easiest feeding challenges.

They're the ones who lean into this work.

Who answer the questions honestly.

Who complete the exercises.

Who are willing to grow right alongside their child.

Those are the families who often move through our program the fastest.

Not because they become perfect.

Because they become different.

That's why this section of the book is about you.

Not because you're the problem.

> Because you're the secret weapon that takes everything to the next level.

The strategies you've learned so far matter.

The Mealtime Agreements matter.

Everything you've put into place matters.

But when those strategies are paired with a parent who is calmer...

More confident...

More patient...

More curious...

Everything changes.

So, buckle up.

Grab a pen.

Keep an open mind.

And promise yourself one thing.

Don't just read the next few chapters.

Do them.

Because I have a feeling that when you reach the final page of this book...

You won't just look at your child's progress.

You'll look in the mirror...

And realize you've changed too.

And that...

May be the greatest gift this journey gives you.

Key Takeaways

- Children don't grow in isolation—they grow within relationships.

- Your mindset influences the emotional environment around every meal.

- The greatest transformation in our program often isn't the child—it's the parent.

- Your child may be one of your greatest teachers.

- You are not the problem.

- You are the secret weapon that takes everything to the next level.

Action Steps

29. Commit to doing every exercise in Part III— even the ones that feel uncomfortable.

30. Before reading the next chapter, ask yourself:

"If this journey changes me just as much as it changes my child... what kind of parent do I hope to become?"

31. Write your answer down.

At the end of this book, come back and read it again. You might be surprised by just how far you've come.

Before We Continue...

The next section of this book is different. You're not just going to read it.

You're going to experience it.

Throughout the remaining chapters, I'll be inviting you to reflect, write, notice patterns, and complete exercises that have helped hundreds of parents transform not only their mealtimes, but also the way they think about feeding.

Because of that, I've created a companion workbook for you. It's completely free.

Inside you'll find every exercise from the rest of this book, along with extra space to reflect, journal, and track your progress.

I encourage you to download it now before moving on to the next chapter. Keep it nearby as you read. Write in it. Highlight it. Come back to it.

These aren't busy-work exercises. They're part of the process.

The parents who lean into this work—the ones who actually complete the exercises instead of simply reading them—are often the ones who experience the biggest transformations.

Scan the code below to download your free copy of The Mealtime Mindset Companion Workbook:

Then grab a pen... **and let's get to work.**

CHAPTER ELEVEN

Training Your Brain

Before You Read...

I want you to try something.

Look around the room you're sitting in and count how many blue things you can find.

Go ahead.

I'll wait.

...

Done?

Now close your eyes.

How many red things were in the room?

Most people have no idea.

Not because there weren't any red things.

Because your brain wasn't looking for them.

Now open your eyes and look for red.

Suddenly...

They're everywhere.

The red logo.

The book spine.

The coffee mug.

The blanket.

The pen.

They were there the entire time.

Your brain simply decided they weren't important.

Your child's feeding journey works exactly the same way.

Your Brain Finds What You Tell It to Find

Your brain has an incredible filtering system.

It decides what deserves your attention.

That means if you spend every meal thinking,

> *"They only eat bread."*

> *"They never sit."*

> *"Nothing is working."*

Guess what your brain is going to notice?

Every bite they didn't take.

Every refusal.

Every setback.

Every hard moment.

But here's the problem.

When your brain is busy collecting evidence that nothing is changing…

It misses the tiny moments that actually matter.

The extra minute they stayed seated.

The new food they tolerated on the plate.

The calmer meal.

The fact that you stayed calm.

Progress doesn't always shout. Most of the time, it whispers.

The Stories We Tell Ourselves

Our thoughts are powerful.

Whether you believe they shape reality, influence your actions, or simply determine what your brain notices...

One thing is certain.

The stories we tell ourselves matter.

If you keep repeating,

> *"Nothing ever changes."*

Your brain will work incredibly hard to prove you right.

What if...

Instead...

You started telling yourself a different story?

> Instead of *"My child only eats bread."*
> Try *"My child is learning to expand their diet."*
>
> Instead of *"They'll never sit at the table."*
> Try *"My child is learning how to eat meals with the family."*

Notice something.

We're not lying.

We're not pretending.

We're acknowledging something incredibly important.

Learning is a process.

Flip the Thought

Open your workbook.

Create three columns.

Write down every negative thought you catch yourself thinking.

Don't censor yourself.

Get them all out.

Examples:

"My child will never eat vegetables."

"This isn't working."

"I'm failing."

Now rewrite each thought.

Not with toxic positivity.

With possibility.

Instead of *"My child hates vegetables."*
Try *"My child is still learning about vegetables."*

Instead of *"We never have good meals."*
Try *"We're learning how to create calmer meals."*

One word can completely change the direction of your thinking.

Now comes the challenge.

Find three things you're grateful for.

Not because everything is wonderful.

Because gratitude teaches your brain to notice what's already going well.

Maybe...

> *"I'm grateful I found this book."*

> *"I'm grateful my child is healthy enough to learn."*

> *"I'm grateful we're working on this now instead of five years from now."*

> *"I'm grateful I know what to do next."*

Some days...

This will be hard.

Do it anyway.

The Future Gratitude Exercise

Now I want to stretch you a little.

Turn the page in your workbook.

Write a date one year from today.

At the top of the page write:

> *I am so grateful that...*

Then write twenty statements.

Write them as though they've already happened.

Not because you're pretending.

Because you're giving your brain something hopeful to work toward.

Maybe...

"I am so grateful family dinners are peaceful."

"I am grateful my child enjoys birthday parties."

"I am grateful restaurants aren't stressful anymore."

"I am grateful my child asks to help cook."

Then...

Don't stop there.

For every statement...

Ask yourself...

Why does this matter?

"I am grateful my child enjoys birthday parties... because now they feel included."

"I am grateful we can go to restaurants... because we make memories instead of worrying."

"I am grateful my child eats more foods... because they have confidence."

See what just happened?

You stopped thinking about broccoli.

And started thinking about life.

Gratitude Changes More Than Your Mood

Gratitude isn't pretending everything is perfect.

It's refusing to let the difficult moments become the only moments you see.

After working with hundreds of families...

I've noticed something.

The parents who intentionally practice gratitude...

Who celebrate tiny wins...

Who notice small shifts...

Who flip negative thoughts...

Those parents often stay motivated longer.

They remain hopeful.

They keep showing up.

And because they keep showing up...

Their children continue making progress.

MINDSET CHALLENGE #2

The Seven-Day Reset

For the next seven days, every night, write down:

> Three wins.
>
> Three things you're grateful for.
>
> One negative thought you flipped.

It'll take less than five minutes. But I think you'll be amazed at what happens—not because your child suddenly changes overnight, but because you begin seeing the journey differently.

And remember...

The greatest transformation often isn't your child's. It's yours.

CHAPTER TWELVE

Releasing Guilt and Self-Blame

Before You Read...

Open your workbook.

At the top of a blank page, write:

> *What do I blame myself for?*

Don't overthink it.

Just write.

Maybe it's...

> *"Maybe I shouldn't have let them eat in front of the TV."*

> *"Maybe I gave them too many pouches."*

> *"I should have noticed this sooner."*

> *"I shouldn't have made a second meal."*

> *"Maybe I pressured them too much."*

> *"Maybe I didn't push enough."*

Whatever comes to mind...

Write it down.

No one else will read it.

This is simply an opportunity to get those thoughts out of your head and onto paper.

When you're finished...

Come back.

Every Parent I've Ever Met

If there's one emotion almost every parent brings into feeding therapy...

It's guilt.

Sometimes it's quiet.

Sometimes it's overwhelming.

But it's almost always there.

Parents wonder...

> *"Did I cause this?"*

> *"If I had done things differently, would we even be here?"*

> *"How did I miss this?"*

Maybe you've wondered the same thing.

Can I tell you something?

I've never met a parent who intentionally created feeding challenges for their child.

Never.

I've met parents who were exhausted.

Parents who were scared.

Parents who were overwhelmed.

Parents who were simply trying to get through the day.

But I've never met one who woke up and thought,

> *"I hope I create a picky eater."*

Every decision you've made has been based on the knowledge, energy, resources, and support you had available at the time.

That's what parenting is.

We're all doing the best we can...

Until we know better.

Then we do better.

Hindsight Is a Wonderful Teacher

One of the hardest parts about becoming a parent is this:

You don't get to learn the lesson...

Until after you've already lived through it.

Looking back, it's easy to think,

> *"I should have known."*

Of course it is.

You're looking backward with today's knowledge.

But yesterday's version of you didn't have today's knowledge.

She was doing the best she could with what she knew at the time.

Expecting your past self to know what your present self knows isn't fair.

It's like expecting your five-year-old to solve algebra.

They simply don't have the information yet.

Neither did you.

Guilt Keeps You Looking in the Wrong Direction

Imagine driving somewhere you've never been before.

Halfway through the trip, you realize you've taken a wrong turn.

Do you spend the rest of the drive staring in the rearview mirror?

Of course not.

You acknowledge it.

Take the next turn.

And keep moving toward your destination.

Guilt has a funny way of keeping us staring into the rearview mirror.

Replaying conversations.

Replaying decisions.

Replaying all the things we wish we had done differently.

> **Your child's progress isn't behind you. It's in front of you.**

The energy you spend reliving the past is energy you can't use creating change today.

Speak to Yourself Like You Would a Friend

Imagine your closest friend called you tomorrow.

She was crying.

Her child was struggling with eating.

She said,

"I think this is all my fault."

What would you say?

Would you tell her,

> *"You're right. You completely ruined your child."*

Of course not.

You'd remind her that she was doing her best.

You'd encourage her.

You'd hug her.

You'd help her see the hope that she couldn't see herself.

Now here's my question.

Why are you deserving of any less compassion?

Your Child Needs Today's Version of You

One of the biggest problems with guilt is that it quietly changes the way we parent.

Parents begin making decisions from fear instead of confidence.

They second-guess every choice.

They become afraid of making another mistake.

Children are incredibly sensitive to this.

They may not know exactly what you're thinking.

But they can often feel when you're anxious, uncertain, or carrying the weight of self-blame.

The parent your child needs today isn't a perfect parent.

They need the parent who's willing to learn.

Who's willing to grow.

Who's willing to try again.

And that's exactly what you're doing.

You're here.

Reading this book.

Showing up.

Learning.

That tells me everything I need to know about the kind of parent you are.

One More Thought…

Earlier in this book, I told you that I believe our children are some of our greatest teachers.

I still believe that.

As difficult as this journey may feel…

I also believe it's shaping you.

Teaching you.

Stretching you.

Helping you become a calmer, more confident, more compassionate parent.

Not someday.

Right now.

The feeding challenges may not be something you would have chosen.

But I have watched them become the catalyst for incredible growth in hundreds of families.

Maybe…

Just maybe...

That can be true for yours too.

The Self-Compassion Rewrite

Go back to the list you wrote at the beginning of this chapter. Next to each statement, write:

> *"At the time, I made the best decision I could with the knowledge, energy, and resources I had."*

Then write one more sentence at the bottom of the page:

> *"Today I know more. And because I know more, I can choose differently moving forward."*

Notice the difference. We're not erasing the past. We're simply refusing to live there.

"You don't need to be the parent who got everything right. You only need to be the parent who's willing to keep learning."

CHAPTER THIRTEEN

Practicing Patience and Trust

Growing the Roots You Can't See

Before You Read...

Grab your workbook.

Before you turn the page, answer one simple question.

How will you know this program is working?

Don't overthink it.

Just write the first answer that comes to mind.

Maybe you wrote:

"My child eats vegetables."

"They finally finish dinner."

"They stop gagging."

"They eat what I cook."

"They'll finally try something new."

Now...

Circle the word that appears in almost every answer.

Eat.

Almost every parent defines success by the final outcome.

And honestly?

That makes perfect sense.

You bought this book because you want your child to eat.

But what if measuring success only by bites is one of the biggest reasons parents lose patience?

The Problem With Measuring the Finish Line

Imagine you signed up to run your very first marathon.

On the first day of training, your coach asks you to jog around the block.

You finish.

Proud of yourself.

Then you throw your hands up and say,

>*"Well... I didn't run twenty-six miles."*

That would sound ridiculous, wouldn't it?

Of course you didn't.

You were building toward it.

No one expects a marathon on Day One.

Yet parents do this with feeding all the time.

A child looks at a new food.

>*"Well... they didn't eat it."*

They touch it.

>*"Still didn't eat it."*

They smell it.

>*"They're still refusing."*

Parents are measuring the finish line…

While completely overlooking the training.

The Bamboo Tree

There's a story I love about the Chinese bamboo tree.

After it's planted, you water it.

You care for it.

You protect it.

Days go by.

Weeks go by.

Months go by.

Sometimes even years.

And…

Nothing.

At least, nothing you can see.

Then one day…

The bamboo suddenly shoots up at an incredible speed.

People often say,

> *"It grew overnight!"*

But that's not what happened at all.

It had been growing the entire time.

Just underground.

Developing an extensive root system strong enough to support the height it was about to reach.

Without those roots…

The tree couldn't survive.

Children often learn about food the same way.

Parents look at the plate and think,

> *"Nothing is happening."*

Meanwhile...

Their child's brain is learning.

Their nervous system is building trust.

Their confidence is growing.

They're collecting safe experiences.

The roots are growing. You just can't see them yet.

Redefining Progress

One of the biggest mindset shifts I hope you'll make after reading this book is this:

Progress is not measured by bites. Progress is measured by learning.

Sometimes learning looks like eating.

But more often...

It looks much smaller.

Progress might look like:

- Looking at a new food.
- Allowing it on the table.
- Letting it stay on the plate.
- Smelling it.

- Touching it.
- Talking about it.
- Staying calm while it's nearby.
- Recovering more quickly after feeling overwhelmed.
- Sitting at the table for a few extra minutes.
- You staying calm when things don't go as planned.

Those moments matter.

In fact...

Those moments are often the very things that eventually lead to eating.

Trust the Process

Patience doesn't mean doing nothing while you wait for your child to "get over it."

Patience is active.

It means continuing to show up.

Continuing to offer opportunities without pressure.

Continuing to follow your Mealtime Agreements.

Continuing to trust that your child is learning, even when you can't see dramatic changes yet.

Every calm meal.

Every predictable routine.

Every safe experience.

Is another root growing beneath the surface.

And every time you respond with patience instead of panic...

You're sending your child a powerful message:

"You're safe."

"I trust you."

Children grow remarkably well in environments where they feel trusted.

When Progress Feels Slow

There will be days when it feels like nothing is changing.

I've had those conversations with parents many times.

They'll tell me,

"We're doing everything you said, but nothing's happening."

Then we start talking.

I ask a few questions.

And suddenly they realize...

The meltdowns have decreased.

Their child is sitting longer.

They're touching foods they never touched before.

Meals feel calmer.

Parents are calmer.

Something has changed.

They just weren't measuring it.

Remember...

If you only measure the final bite...

You'll miss all the roots growing underneath.

Rewrite the Finish Line

Go back to the goal you wrote at the beginning of this chapter. Now rewrite it.

Instead of writing the finish line, write the skills your child needs to build to get there. For example:

Instead of *"My child eats vegetables."*

Try *"My child is learning to feel safe around vegetables."*

Or "My child is becoming more curious about vegetables."

Or "My child is building the confidence to explore vegetables."

Notice how different that feels. One creates pressure. The other creates possibility.

Keep this new version somewhere you'll see it often. Let it become the way you measure progress moving forward.

Key Takeaways

- Patience isn't passive. It's choosing to show up consistently with calm confidence.

- Progress is not measured by bites. It's measured by learning.

- The most important growth often happens before you can see it.

- Children need strong roots before they can grow.

- Trust the process, even when the progress feels quiet.

CHAPTER FOURTEEN

You're Part of the Story

Before You Read...

Open your workbook.

I have two questions for you.

The first one is easy.

> *If your feeding journey were a book... what would the title be?*

Don't overthink it.

Just write whatever comes to mind.

Maybe it's...

> *The Never-Ending Battle.*
>
> *One More Bite.*
>
> *Dinner Wars.*
>
> *The Child Who Wouldn't Eat.*

Or maybe...

> *Learning Together.*

Now for the second question.

> *Who is the main character?*

Your child?

You?

Your whole family?

Write your answer down before you continue.

A Story We All Tell

One of the most fascinating things I've learned is that human beings naturally make sense of life through stories.

When something difficult happens, our brains instinctively begin asking questions.

"Why is this happening?"

"Who is this happening to?"

"How does it end?"

Stories help us organize experiences.

They help us make meaning out of moments that otherwise feel confusing.

The problem is...

We don't just tell stories about books and movies.

We tell stories about ourselves.

About our children.

About our families.

Sometimes those stories become so familiar that we stop questioning them.

"My child is just a picky eater."

"We've always struggled."

"Dinner is always a battle."

"My child doesn't eat strawberries."

Those statements begin to feel like facts.

But are they?

Or are they simply the story you've been telling yourself?

The Power of "Yet"

Let's go back to strawberries for a moment.

Listen to the difference between these two sentences.

> *"My child doesn't eat strawberries."*

Now try this one.

> *"My child hasn't learned enough about strawberries yet to feel comfortable eating them regularly."*

Do you feel the difference?

The first sentence closes the book.

The second one leaves another chapter to be written.

It acknowledges something incredibly important.

Learning takes time.

Comfort takes experience.

Growth is still happening.

The story isn't over.

It's Not Just Your Child's Story

Here's something that surprises almost every parent who goes through our program.

They begin believing this journey is about changing their child.

After all...

Their child is the one refusing food.

Their child is the one gagging.

Their child is the one melting down.

So naturally they think,

> *"I'm just here to help my child."*

But somewhere along the way...

Something unexpected happens.

They begin to change too.

They become calmer.

More confident.

More patient.

They communicate differently.

They understand their child differently.

They enjoy mealtimes more.

And one day they realize...

> *"This wasn't just my child's story."*

> *"It was mine too."*

Finding Nemo

Think about the movie Finding Nemo.

Most people assume it's Nemo's story.

After all...

His name is in the title.

He's the one who gets lost.

He's the one who needs rescuing.

But by the end of the movie...

Who changed the most?

Marlin.

He began the story fearful.

Controlling.

Convinced the world wasn't safe.

He believed protecting Nemo meant never letting him struggle.

As the story unfolded, Nemo grew more independent.

But Marlin grew too.

He learned trust.

He learned courage.

He learned to let go.

The story didn't transform just one character.

It transformed them both.

Your feeding journey is remarkably similar.

You may have picked up this book because you wanted to help your child.

And I hope you do.

But my hope is something else happens too.

I hope somewhere along this journey...

You discover you've changed as well.

Our Stories Grow Together

One of the greatest lessons this work has taught me is this:

Children and parents grow together.

As your child becomes more curious...

You become more patient.

As your child builds confidence...

You begin trusting the process.

As your child learns flexibility...

You begin letting go of fear.

Neither journey happens in isolation.

Your stories are intertwined.

One person's growth creates space for the other's.

I've seen this happen hundreds of times.

Parents come to us hoping their child will change.

They leave amazed by the person they've become.

Maybe This Challenge Is Teaching You Too

I truly believe our children are some of our greatest teachers.

As much as we guide them...

They shape us.

This feeding journey may be teaching your child about food.

But perhaps it's also teaching you...

Patience.

Trust.

Compassion.

Boundaries.

Curiosity.

Resilience.

Maybe this challenge entered your life for more than one reason.

Maybe there was something here for both of you to learn.

MINDSET CHALLENGE #5

Write the Ending

Turn to the next page in your workbook. At the top, write:

The Final Chapter

Imagine it's one year from now. Someone asks,

"Tell me the story of your feeding journey."

How does it end? Not "What foods does your child eat?"—tell me the story.

Who did your child become? Who did you become? How did your relationship change? What did this experience teach your family?

Write it in the past tense, as though you've already lived it. Don't worry about getting it perfect. Just write.

Because here's something I hope you remember.

You're not reading the last chapter of your story. You're still writing it.

Key Takeaways

We naturally understand life through stories.

The stories we tell ourselves shape how we see our child and ourselves.

"Yet" keeps the story open to growth.

This feeding journey isn't just changing your child.

It's changing you too.

Children and parents grow together.

Their stories are intertwined.

- The chapter you're living today doesn't get to decide how the story ends.

. . .

One Last Thing...

If you've made it this far, I want you to pause for a moment.

Think back to the parent who opened this book.

The one who felt exhausted.

Frustrated.

Maybe guilty.

Maybe wondering if anything would ever change.

Now think about the parent reading these words.

You may not have transformed your child's eating overnight.

But I hope something else has already begun to change.

The way you see your child.

The way you see yourself.

The way you see mealtimes.

Because once your perspective changes...

Everything else begins to change with it.

You'll notice opportunities where you used to see obstacles.

You'll respond with curiosity instead of fear.

You'll recognize progress that once went unnoticed.

You'll stop measuring success by one bite...

...and start measuring it by one brave step.

And those steps add up.

One day, your child may sit down and happily eat something they once refused.

That day will feel incredible.

But I have a feeling something else will surprise you even more.

You'll realize...

You changed too.

You'll be calmer.

More confident.

More patient.

More connected.

You'll know exactly what to say—and when saying nothing is actually the better choice.

You'll trust yourself.

And your child will begin trusting themselves too.

Remember what we talked about?

This was never just your child's story.

It was yours.

Your stories have been intertwined from the very beginning.

As you changed...

They changed.

As they grew...

So did you.

That is the beautiful thing about parenting.

Our children don't just learn from us.

They transform us.

So keep going.

Celebrate the tiny victories.

Stay curious.

Trust the process.

And whenever the journey feels hard...

Come back to one simple question.

What story do I want to help write today?

Because every meal...

Every conversation...

Every tiny moment of connection...

Is another sentence in your family's story.

Make it one worth telling.

. . .

Before You Go...

Don't forget to download your FREE Mealtime Mindset™ Companion Workbook.

Inside you'll find all of the exercises from this book, along with printable worksheets, trackers, reflection prompts, and action steps to help you put these ideas into practice.

You can download it here:

Scan to download

And if this book encouraged you, I have one small favor to ask.

Would you consider leaving an honest review on Amazon?

Your review doesn't just help this book.

It helps another tired parent find hope.

Sometimes all it takes is reading one person's experience to finally believe:

> *"Maybe things can get better for us too."*

Thank you for allowing me to be a small part of your family's story.

I'm cheering for you.

Always.

— Christine